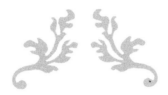

Low-Carb Recipes 2021

The Ultimate Recipes Collection for Easy Low-Carb Recipes
| Try Over 50 Mouth-Watering Keto Recipes For Weight
Loss

Albert Lee

Table of Contents

1. Hot Buffalo Wings

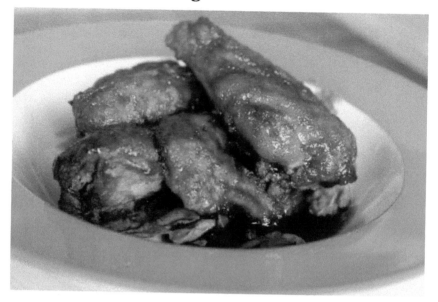

Serving: 8

Prep Time: 10 minutes

Cook Time:6 hours

Ingredients

- 1 bottle of (12 ounces) hot pepper sauce
- ½ cup melted ghee
- 1 tablespoon dried oregano + onion powder
- 2 teaspoons garlic powder
- 5 pounds chicken wing sections

How To

1. Take a large bowl and mix in hot sauce, ghee, garlic powder, oregano, onion powder, and mix well

2. Add chicken wings and toss to coat

3. Pour mix into Slow Cooker and cook on LOW for 6 hours

4. Serve and enjoy!

Nutrition (Per Serving)

- Calories: 529
- Fat: 4g
- Carbohydrates: 1g
- Protein: 31g

Tip: If you don't have a slow cooker, you may use an Iron-Cast Dutch Oven. The temperature is 200 Degrees F for LOW and 250 degrees F for HIGH

2. A Jar Full Of Pecans

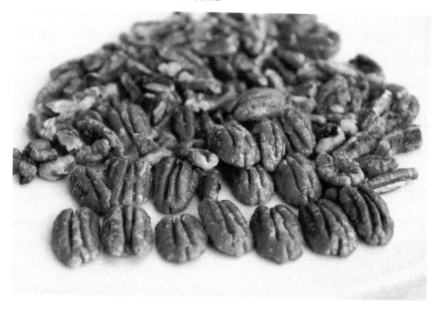

Serving: 4

Prep Time: 10 minutes

Cook Time:2 hours

Ingredients

- 3 cups of raw pecans
- ¼ cup of date paste
- 2 teaspoon of vanilla beans extract
- 1 teaspoon of sea salt
- 1 tablespoon of coconut oil

How To

1. Add all of the listed ingredients to your pot

2. Cook on LOW for about 3 hours, making sure to stir it from time to time

3. Once done, allow it to cool and serve!

Nutrition (Per Serving)

- Calories: 337
- Fat: 31g
- Carbohydrates: 16g
- Protein: 4g

3. The Exquisite Spaghetti Squash

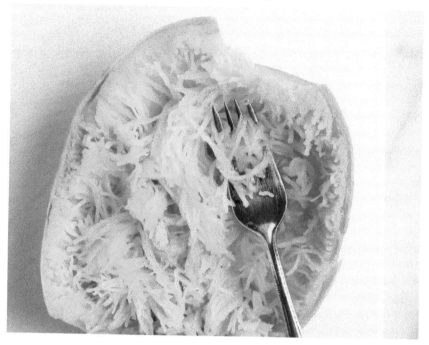

Serving: 6

Prep Time: 5 minutes

Cook Time: 7-8 hours

Ingredients

- 1 spaghetti squash
- 2 cups water

How To

1. Wash squash carefully with water and rinse it well

2. Puncture 5-6 holes in the squash using a fork

3. Place squash in Slow Cooker

4. Place lid and cook on LOW for 7-8 hours

5. Remove squash to a cutting board and let it cool

6. Cut squash in half and discard seeds

7. Use two forks and scrape out squash strands and transfer to the bowl

8. Serve and enjoy!

Nutrition (Per Serving)

- Calories: 52
- Fat: 0g
- Carbohydrates: 12g
- Protein: 1g

Tip: If you don't have a slow cooker, you may use an Iron-Cast Dutch Oven. The temperature is 200 Degrees F for LOW and 250 degrees F for HIGH

4. Worthy Bacon-Wrapped Drumsticks

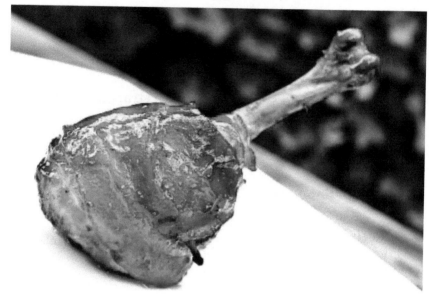

Serving: 6

Prep Time: 10 minutes

Cook Time:8 hours

Ingredients

- 12 chicken drumsticks
- 12 slices thin-cut bacon

How To

1. Wrap each chicken drumsticks in bacon

2. Place drumsticks in your Slow Cooker

3. Place lid and cook on LOW for 8 hours

4. Serve and enjoy!

Nutrition (Per Serving)

- Calories: 202
- Fat: 8g
- Carbohydrates: 3g
- Protein: 30g

Tip: If you don't have a slow cooker, you may use an Iron-Cast Dutch Oven. The temperature is 200 Degrees F for LOW and 250 degrees F for HIGH

5. Coconut Chocolate Cookie

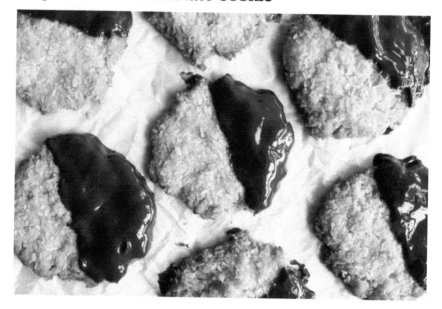

Serving: 4

Prep Time: 10 minutes

Cook Time: Nil

<u>Ingredients</u>

- 4 cups unsweetened coconut, shredded

- ½ cup coconut milk

- ¼ cup sugar-free maple syrup

- ¼ teaspoon almond extract

How To

1. Blend coconut in your food processor until you have a nice texture.

2. Add coconut milk and syrup; keep blending until you have a nice batter.

3. Add more milk if the batter is a bit too crumbly.

4. Transfer the mixture to the mixing bowl.

5. Use your hand to form small balls.

6. Line a baking tray with parchment paper and transfer the balls, flatten them lightly to form a cookie shape.

7. Sprinkle coconut on top and chill for 2-3 hour until firm

8. Enjoy!

Nutrition (Per Serving)

- Calories: 40
- Fat: 4g
- Carbohydrates: 2g
- Protein: 1g

6. Keto Shortbread

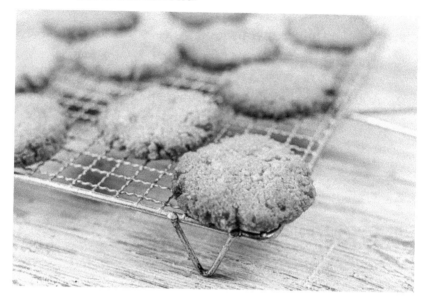

Serving: 4

Prep Time: 10 minutes

Cook Time: 15 minutes

Ingredients

- ½ cup Erythritol

- 1 teaspoon vanilla extract

- 2 and ½ cups almond flour

- 6 tablespoons butter

How To

1. Pre-heat your oven to 350 degrees F.

2. Line cookie sheet with parchment paper.

3. Take a bowl and beat in butter, Erythritol and mix until it is fluffy.

4. Beat in vanilla extract, beat in almond flour ½ cup at a time.

5. Use a tablespoon to transfer the dough to a cookie sheet.

6. Flatten each cookie to about 1/3 inch thick.

7. Bake for 12-15 minutes until golden.

8. Let them cool and serve

9. Enjoy!

Nutrition (Per Serving)

- Calories: 124
- Fat: 12g
- Carbohydrates: 2g
- Protein: 3g

7. 1 Minute Keto Muffin

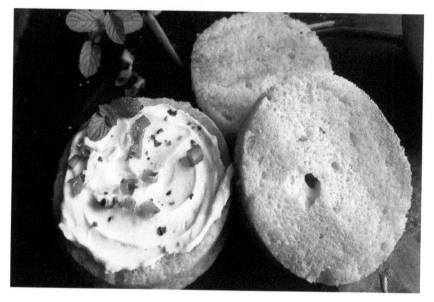

Serving: 4

Prep Time: 10 minutes

Cook Time: 1 minute

Ingredients

- 1 whole egg

- 2 teaspoon coconut flour

- A pinch of baking soda

- A pinch salt

- Coconut oil, for grease

How To

1. Grease ramekin dish with coconut oil.

2. Keep it aside.

3. Take a bowl and add ingredients and mix well.

4. Pour batter into a ramekin.

5. Place into microwave for 1 minute on HIGH.

6. Serve and enjoy!

Nutrition (Per Serving)

- Calories: 102
- Fat: 5g
- Carbohydrates: 3g
- Protein: 7g

8. Chilled No-Bake Lemon Cheesecake

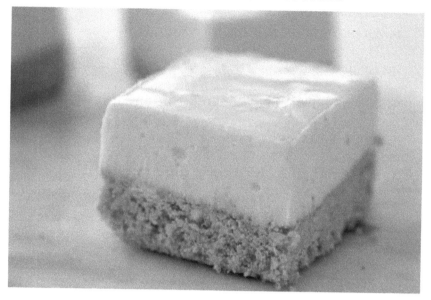

Serving: 4

Prep Time: 10 minutes + 60 minutes Chill Time

Cook Time: Nil

<u>Ingredients</u>

- 6-8 ounces cream cheese

- 2 ounces full-fat cream

- 1 tablespoon lemon juice

- Few drops of vanilla extract

- Peel ½ lemon, grated

How To

1. Add cream, cream cheese, and mix well.

2. Add the remaining ingredients.

3. Transfer the mixture to your fridge.

4. Keep it for 1 hour in the fridge.

5. Serve and enjoy!

Nutrition (Per Serving)

- Calories: 220
- Fat: 17g
- Carbohydrates: 2g
- Protein: 6g

9. Delicious Vegetable Quiche

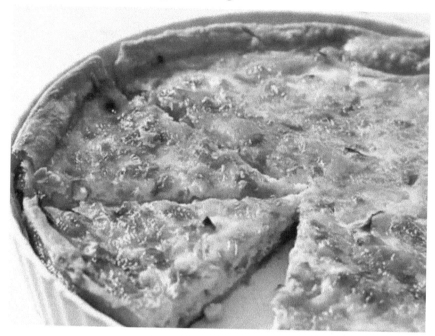

Serving: 4

Prep Time: 10 minutes

Cook Time: 25 minutes

<u>Ingredients</u>

- 1 tablespoon melted butter, divided
- 6 eggs
- 3 ounces (85 g) goat cheese, divided
- 3/4 cup heavy whipping cream
- 1 scallion, white and green parts, chopped
- 1/2 cup mushrooms, sliced

- 1 cup fresh spinach, chopped
- 10 cherry tomatoes, cut in half

How To

1. Preheat the oven to 350°F (180°C). Coat a pie pan with 1/2 teaspoon of melted butter and set aside.

2. Whisk together the eggs, 2 ounces (57 g) of goat cheese, and heavy whipping cream in a bowl until creamy and smooth, you can use a blender to make it easier. Set aside.

3. Heat the remaining butter in a nonstick skillet over medium-high heat. Add and saute scallion and mushrooms for 2 minutes or until tender. Add and saute the spinach for another 2 minutes or until softened.

4. Pour the vegetable mixture into the pie pan, and use a spatula to spread the mixture so it covers the bottom of the pan evenly.

5. Pour the egg mixture over the vegetable mixture. Top them with the cherry tomato halves and remaining goat cheese.

6. Place the pie pan in the preheated oven and bake for 20 minutes or until fluffy. You can check the doneness by cutting a small slit in the center, if raw eggs run into the cut, then baking for another few minutes.

7. Divide the quiche among four platters and serve warm.

<u>Nutrition (Per Serving)</u>

- Calories: 395
- Fat: 32g
- Carbohydrates: 4g
- Protein: 21g

10.   Fancy Rutabaga Cakes

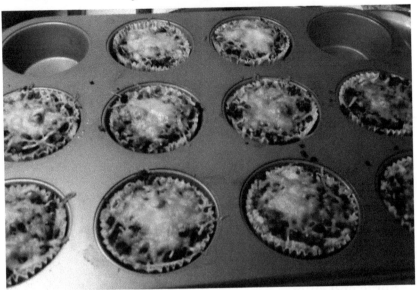

Serving: 4

Prep Time: 10 minutes

Cook Time: 25-30 minutes

Ingredients

- 2 rutabagas, thinly sliced

- ½ stick butter, melted

- 2 tablespoons fresh thyme, chopped

- 2 teaspoons salt

How To

1. Place a saucepan over medium heat.

2. Add butter and let it melt.

3. Add thyme and stir for 2 minutes.

4. Take a bowl and add rutabaga slices into it and pour the mix.

5. Layer rutabaga slices in muffin tins and top with butter on top.

6. Take a foil and cover muffin tins.

7. Preheat your oven to 350 degrees F.

8. Bake for 25-30 minutes.

9. Serve and enjoy!

Nutrition (Per Serving)

- Calories: 46
- Fat: 3g
- Carbohydrates: 1g
- Protein: 0.4g

11. Eggplant Fries

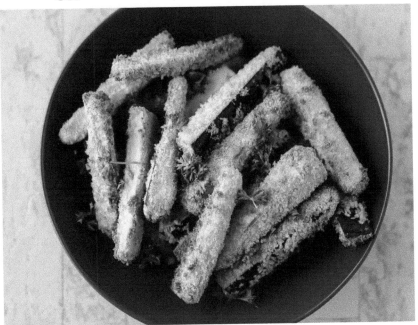

Serving: 4

Prep Time: 10 minutes

Cook Time: 15 minutes

<u>Ingredients</u>

- 2 whole eggs

- 2 cups almond flour

- 2 tablespoons coconut oil, spray

- 2 eggplant, peeled and cut thinly

- Salt and pepper to taste

How To

1. Preheat your oven to 400 degrees Fahrenheit.

2. Take a bowl and mix with salt and black pepper in it.

3. Take another bowl and beat eggs until frothy.

4. Dip the eggplant pieces into eggs.

5. Then coat them with a flour mixture.

6. Add another layer of flour and egg.

7. Then, take a baking sheet and grease with coconut oil on top.

8. Bake for about 15 minutes.

9. Serve and enjoy!

Nutrition (Per Serving)

- Calories: 212
- Fat: 15g
- Carbohydrates: 4g
- Protein: 7g

12. Stuffed Parmesan Cheese Avocado

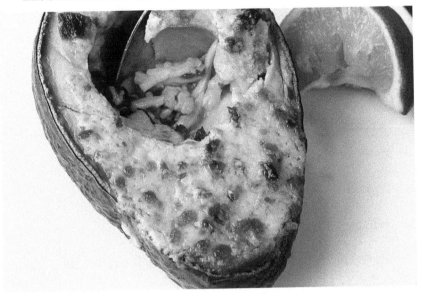

Serving: 4

Prep Time: 10 minutes

Cook Time: 15 minutes

Ingredients

- 1 whole avocado

- 1 tablespoon chipotle sauce

- 1 tablespoon lime juice

- ¼ cup parmesan cheese

- Salt and pepper to taste

How To

1. Prepare avocado by slicing half lengthwise and discard the seed.

2. Gently prick the skin of the avocado with a fork.

3. Set your avocado halves, skin down on the small baking sheet lined with aluminum foil.

4. Top with sauce and drizzle lime juice.

5. Season with salt and pepper.

6. Sprinkle half parmesan cheese in each cavity, set your broiler to high for 2 minutes.

7. Add rest of the cheese and return to your broiler until cheese melts and avocado slightly browns.

8. Serve hot and enjoy!

Nutrition (Per Serving)

- Calories: 41
- Fat: 41g
- Carbohydrates: 7g
- Protein: 7g

13. Orange And Coconut Creamsicles

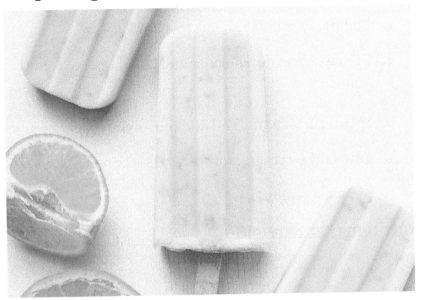

Serving: 4

Prep Time: 10 minutes + 3 Hours Chill Time

Cook Time: Nil

<u>Ingredients</u>

- A ½ cup of coconut oil

- ½ cup heavy whipping cream

- 4 ounces cream cheese

- 1 teaspoon orange mix

- 10 drops liquid stevia

How To

1. Add the listed ingredients to a bowl.

2. Use an immersion blender and blend the mixture well.

3. Take a silicone tray and add the mixture.

4. Keep in the refrigerator for 2-3 hours.

5. Serve and enjoy!

Nutrition (Per Serving)

- Calories: 176
- Fat: 20g
- Carbohydrates: 0.5g
- Protein: 0.8g

14.Coffee Popsicles

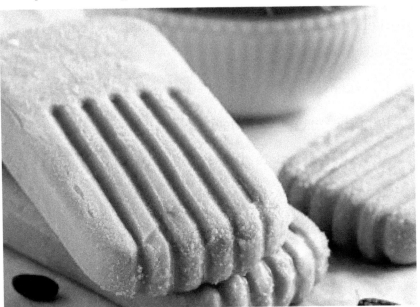

Serving: 4

Prep Time: 10 minutes

Cook Time: Nil

Ingredients

- 2 tablespoons chocolate chips, sugar-free
- 2 cups coffee, brewed and cold
- ¾ cup heavy whip cream
- 2 teaspoons natural sweetener

How To

1. Blend in heavy whip cream, sweetened, and coffee in your blender.

2. Mix them well.

3. Pour the mix into popsicle molds.

4. Add a few chocolate chips.

5. Keep in the fridge for 2 hours.

6. Serve and enjoy!

Nutrition (Per Serving)

- Calories: 105
- Fat: 10g
- Carbohydrates: 2g
- Protein: 2g

15. Icy Berry Popsicles

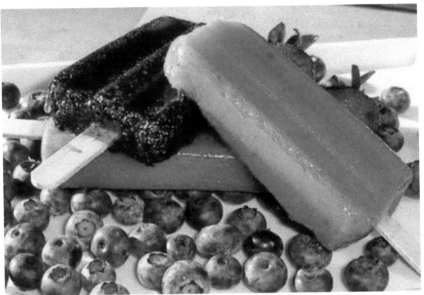

Serving: 4

Prep Time: 10 minutes + 2 Hours Chill Time

Cook Time: Nil

<u>Ingredients</u>

- ¼ cup mixed blackberries and blueberries
- 2 cups coconut cream
- 2 teaspoons stevia

<u>How To</u>

1. Blend the listed ingredients into your blender.

2. Blend until smooth.

3. Pour the mix into popsicle molds.

4. Keep in the fridge for 2 hours.

5. Serve and enjoy!

Nutrition (Per Serving)

- Calories: 165
- Fat: 17g
- Carbohydrates: 3g
- Protein: 1g

16. Scrambled Pesto Eggs

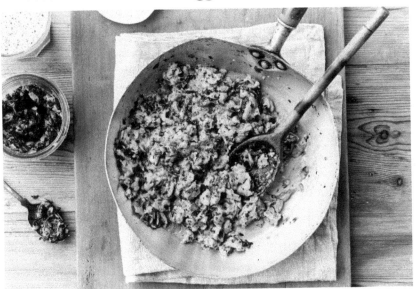

Serving: 4

Prep Time: 5 minutes

Cook Time: 5 minutes

Ingredients

- 3 large whole eggs
- 1 tablespoon butter
- 1 tablespoon pesto
- 2 tablespoons creamed coconut milk
- Salt and pepper as needed

How To

1. Take a bowl and crack open your egg

2. Season with a pinch of salt and pepper

3. Pour eggs into a pan

4. Add butter and introduce heat

5. Cook on low heat and gently add pesto

6. Once the egg is cooked and scrambled, remove heat

7. Spoon in coconut cream and mix well

8. Turn on the heat and cook on LOW for a while until you have a creamy texture

9. Serve and enjoy!

Nutrition (Per Serving)

- Calories: 467
- Fat: 41g
- Carbohydrates: 3g
- Protein: 20g

17. Black Berry Chicken Wings

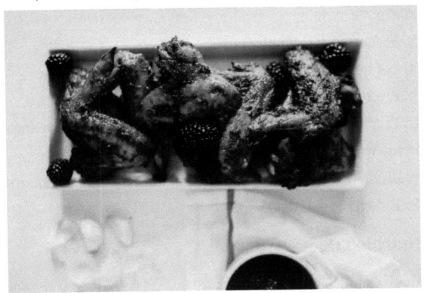

Serving: 4

Prep Time: 35 minutes

Cook Time: 50minutes

Ingredients

- 3 pounds chicken wings, about 20 pieces
- ½ cup blackberry chipotle jam
- Salt and pepper to taste
- ½ cup water

How To

1. Add water and jam to a bowl and mix well

2. Place chicken wings in a zip bag and add two-thirds of the marinade

3. Season with salt and pepper

4. Let it marinate for 30 minutes

5. Pre-heat your oven to 400 degrees F

6. Prepare a baking sheet and wire rack, place chicken wings in the wire rack and bake for 15 minutes

7. Brush remaining marinade and bake for 30 minutes more

8. Enjoy!

<u>Nutrition (Per Serving)</u>

- Calories: 502
- Fat: 39g
- Carbohydrates: 01.8g
- Protein: 34g

18.Awesome Asian Beef Steak

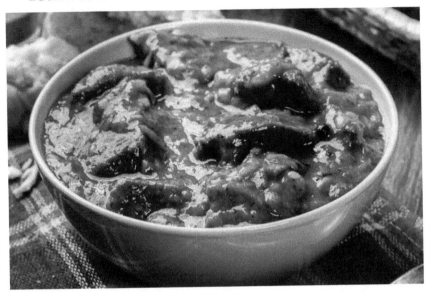

Serving: 3

Prep Time: 10 minutes

Cook Time: 5 minutes

<u>Ingredients</u>

- 2 tablespoon of sriracha sauce
- 1 tablespoon of garlic, minced
- 1 tablespoon of ginger, freshly grated
- 1 yellow bell pepper, cut in strips
- 1 red bell pepper cut in thin strips
- 1 tablespoon of sesame oil, garlic flavored
- 1 tablespoon of stevia

- ½ a teaspoon of curry powder
- ½ a teaspoon of rice wine vinegar
- 8 ounce of beef sirloin cut into strips
- 2 cups of baby spinach, stemmed
- ½ head of butter of lettuce, torn

How To

1. Add garlic, sriracha sauce, 1 teaspoon of sesame oil, rice wine vinegar and stevia bowl

2. Mix well

3. Pour half of the mix into zip bag and add steak, allow it to marinade

4. Assemble the brightly colored salad by layer the vegetables in two bowls in the following order: baby spinach, butter lettuce, two peppers on top

5. Remove the steak from marinade and discard the liquid

6. Heat up sesame oil in skillet over medium heat and add steak, stir fry for 3 minutes

7. Transfer your cooker steak on top of the salad

8. Drizzle the other half of your marinade mix

9. Sprinkle sriracha sauce on top and serve!

Nutrition (Per Serving)

- Calories: 350
- Fat: 23g
- Carbohydrates: 4g
- Protein: 28g

19. Healthy Avocado Beef Patties

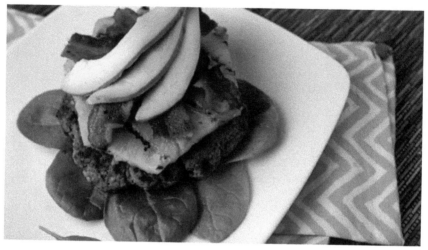

Serving: 2

Prep Time: 15 minutes

Cook Time: 10 minutes

Ingredients

- 1 pound of 85% lean ground beef
- 1 small avocado, pitted and peeled
- 2 slices of yellow cheddar cheese
- Salt as needed
- Fresh ground black pepper as needed

How To

1. Pre-heat and prepare your broiler to high
2. Divide beef into two equal sized patties

3. Season the patties with salt and pepper accordingly
4. Broil the patties for 5 minutes per side
5. Transfer the patties to a platter and add cheese
6. Slice avocado into strips and place them on top of the patties
7. Serve and enjoy!

Nutrition(Per Serving)

- Calories: 568
- Fat: 43g
- Net Carbohydrates: 9g
- Protein: 38g

20.   TheFresh Thai Beef

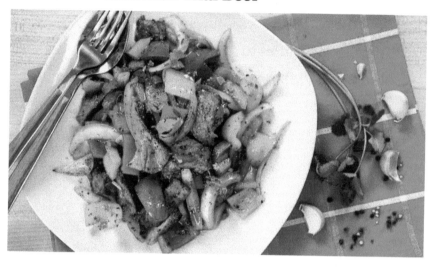

Serving: 4

Prep Time: 10 minutes

Cook Time: 10 minutes

Ingredients

- 1 cup beef stock
- 4 tablespoons peanut butter
- ¼ teaspoon garlic powder
- ¼ teaspoon onion powder
- 1 tablespoon coconut aminos
- 1 and ½ teaspoons lemon pepper
- 1 pound beef steak, cut into strips
- Salt and pepper to taste

- 1 green bell pepper, seeded and chopped
- 3 green onions, chopped

How To

1. Take a bowl and add peanut butter, stock, aminos, lemon pepper and stir

2. Keep the mixture on the side

3. Take a pan and place it over medium-high heat

4. Add beef, season with salt, pepper, onion, garlic powder

5. Cook for 7 minutes

6. Add green pepper, stir cook for 3 minutes

7. Add peanut sauce and green onions

8. Stir cook for 1 minute

9. Divide between platters and serve

10. Enjoy!

Nutrition (Per Serving)

- Calories: 224
- Fat: 15g
- Carbohydrates: 3g
- Protein: 19g

21. Beef Zucchini Chips

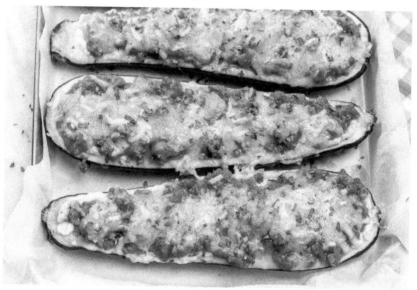

Serving: 4

Prep Time: 10 minutes

Cook Time: 35 minutes

Ingredients

- 2 garlic cloves, peeled and minced
- 1 teaspoon cumin
- 1 tablespoon coconut oil
- 1 pound ground beef
- ½ cup onion, chopped
- 1 teaspoon smoked paprika
- Salt and pepper to taste

- 3 zucchini, sliced lenghtwise, insides scooped out
- ¼ cup fresh cilantro, chopped
- ½ cup cheddar cheese, shredded
- 1 and ½ cups keto-friendly enchilada sauce
- Avocado, chopped
- Green onions, chopped
- Tomatoes, cored and chopped

How To

1. Take a pan and place it over medium-high heat
2. Add oil and heat it up
3. Add onions and stir cook for 2 minutes
4. Add beef and stir for a few minutes
5. Add paprika, salt, pepper, cumin, garlic and stir cook for 2 minutes
6. Transfer zucchini halves to baking pan
7. Stuff each with beef mix, pour enchilada sauce on top
8. Sprinkle cheddar
9. Bake (covered) for 20 minutes at 350-degree F
10. Uncover and sprinkle cilantro
11. Bake for 5 minutes more
12. Sprinkle avocado, green onions, tomatoes on top
13. Serve and enjoy!

Nutrition (Per Serving)

- Calories: 222
- Fat: 10g
- Carbohydrates: 8g
- Protein: 21g

22. Juicy Ground Beef Casserole

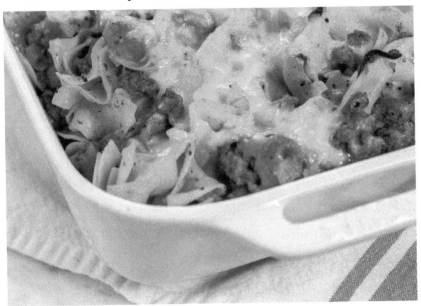

Serving: 6

Prep Time: 10 minutes

Cook Time: 35 minutes

Ingredients

- 2 teaspoons onion flakes
- 1 tablepson glutten-free worcestershire sauce
- 2 pounds ground beef
- 2 garlic clove, peeled and minced
- Salt and pepper to taste
- 1 cup mozarella cheese, shredded
- 2 cups cheddar cheese,shredded

- 1 cup russian dressing
- 2 tablespons sesame seeds, toasted
- 20 dill pickle slices
- 1 romain lettuce head, torn

How To

1. Take a pan and place it over medium heat
2. Add beef, onion flakes, Worcestershire sauce, salt, pepper and garlic
3. Stir for 5 minutes
4. Transfer to baking dish and add a 1 cup of cheddar, mozzarella cheese, half of dressing
5. Stir and spread evenly
6. Arrange pickle slices on top
7. Sprinkle remaining cheddar and sesame seeds
8. Transfer to oven and bake for 20 minutes at 350-degree F
9. Turn oven to broil and broil for 5 minutes
10. Divide lettuce between serving platters and top with remaining dressing
11. Enjoy!

Nutrition (Per Serving)

- Calories: 554
- Fat: 51g
- Carbohydrates: 5g
- Protein: 45g

23. Majestic Beef And Tomato Squash

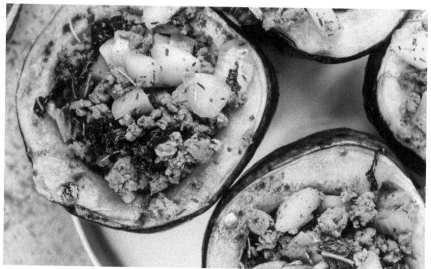

Serving: 4

Prep Time: 10 minutes

Cook Time: 60 minutes

Ingredients

- 2 pounds acorn squash, pricked with fork
- Salt and pepper to taste
- 3 garlic cloves, peeled and minced
- 1 onion, peeled and chopped
- 1 portobello mushroom, sliced
- 28 ounces canned tomatoes, diced
- 1 teaspoon dried oregano
- ¼ teaspoon cayenne pepper

- ½ teaspoon dried thyme
- 1 pound ground beef
- 1 green bell pepper, seeded and chopped

How To

1. Pre-heat your oven to 400 degree F
2. Take acorn squash and transfer to lined baking sheet, bake for 40 minutes
3. Cut in half and let it cool
4. Deseed them
5. Take a pan and place it over medium-high heat, add meat, garlic, onion and mushroom, stir cook until brown
6. Add salt, pepper, thyme, oregano, cayenne, tomatoes, green pepper and stir
7. Cook for 10 minutes
8. Stuff squash halves with beef mix
9. Transfer to oven and bake for 10 minutes more
10. Serve and enjoy!

Nutrition (Per Serving)

- Calories: 260
- Fat: 7g
- Carbohydrates: 4g
- Protein: 10g

24.   Tamari Steak Salad

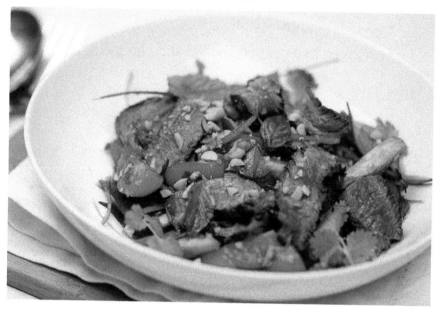

Serving: 4

Prep Time: 15 minutes

Cook Time: 10 minutes

Ingredients

- 2 large bunches salad greens
- 8-9 ounces beef steak
- ½ red bell pepper, siced
- 6-8 cherry tomatoes, cut into halves
- 4 radishes, sliced
- 4 tablespoons olive oil
- ½ tablespoon fresh lemon juice

- 2 ounces gluten free tamari sauce
- Salt as needed

How To

1. Marinate steak in tamari sauce
2. Make salad by adding bell pepper, tomatoes, radishes, salad green, oil, salt and lemon juice to a bowl, and toss them well
3. Grill the steak to your desired doneness and transfer steak on top of the salad platter
4. Let it sit for 1 minute and cut it crosswise
5. Serve and enjoy!

Nutrition (Per Serving)

- Calories: 500
- Fat: 37g
- Carbohydrates: 4g
- Protein: 33g

25.   Ravaging Beef Pot Roast

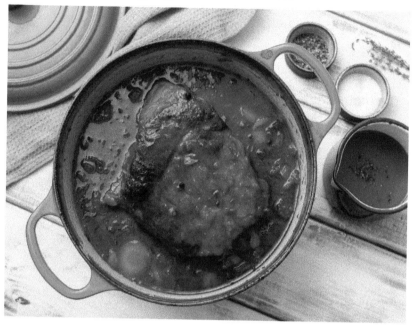

Serving: 4

Prep Time: 10 minutes

Cook Time: 75 minutes

<u>Ingredients</u>

- 3 and ½ pounds beef roast
- 4 ounces mushrooms, sliced
- 12 ounces beef stock
- 1 ounce onion soup mix
- ½ cup Italian dressing

How To

1. Take a bowl and add stock, onion soup mix and Italian dressing

2. Stir

3. Put beef roast in pan

4. Add mushrooms, stock mix to the pan and cover with foil

5. Pre-heat your oven to 300 degree F

6. Bake for 1 hour and 15 minutes

7. Let the roast cool

8. Slice and serve

9. Enjoy with the gravy on top!

Nutrition (Per Serving)

- Calories: 700
- Fat: 56g
- Carbohydrates: 10g
- Protein: 70g

26. Juicy Glazed Beef Meatloaf

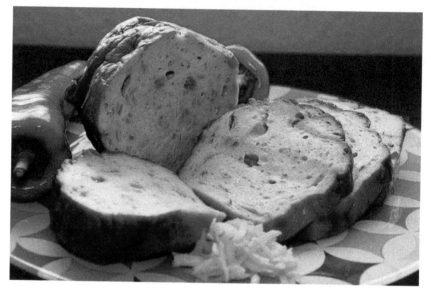

Serving: 6

Prep Time: 10 minutes

Cook Time: 1 hour 10 minutes

Ingredients

- 1 cup white mushrooms, chopped
- 3 pounds ground beef
- 2 tablespoons fresh parsley, chopped
- 2 garlic cloves, peeled and minced
- ½ cup onion, chopped
- ¼ cup red bell pepper, seeded and chopped
- ½ cup almond flour

- 1/3 cup parmesan cheese, grated
- 3 whole eggs
- Salt and pepper to taste
- 1 teaspoon balsamic vinegar

For Glaze

- 1 tablespoon swerve
- 2 tablespoons sugar-free ketchup
- 2 cups balsamic vinegar

How To

1. Take a bowl and add beef, salt, pepper, mushrooms, garlic, onion, bell pepper, parsley, almond flour , cheese, 1 teaspoon vinegar, salt, pepper, eggs and stir well

2. Transfer mixture to loaf pan and bake for 30 minutes at 375 degree F

3. Take a small pan and heat over medium heat

4. Add ketchup, swerve, 2 cups vinegar and stir cook for 20 minutes

5. Take meatloaf out of oven and spread glaze over meatloaf

6. Place in oven and bake for 20 minutes more

7. Let it cool, slice and serve!

<u>Nutrition (Per Serving)</u>

- Calories: 264
- Fat: 14g
- Carbohydrates: 4g
- Protein: 24g

27. Zucchini Beef Sauté With Coriander Greens

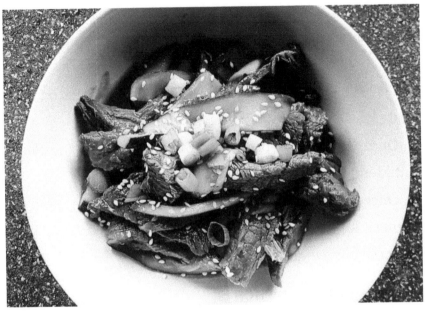

Serving: 4

Prep Time: 10 minutes

Cook Time: 10 minutes

Ingredients

- 10 ounces beef, sliced into 1-2 inch strips
- 1 zuccchini, cut into 2 inch strips
- ¼ cup parsley, chopped
- 3 garlic cloves, minced
- 2 tablespoons tamari sauce

- 4 tablespoons avocado oil

How To

1. Add 2 tablespoons avocado oil in a frying pan over high heat

2. Place strips of beef and brown for a few minutes on high heat

3. Once the meat is brown, add zucchini strips and Saute until tender

4. Once tender, add tamari sauce, garlic, parsley and let them sit for a few minutes more

5. Serve immediately and enjoy!

Nutrition (Per Serving)

- Calories: 500
- Fat: 40g
- Carbohydrates: 5g
- Protein: 31g

28. Pure Broccoli Rib Eye

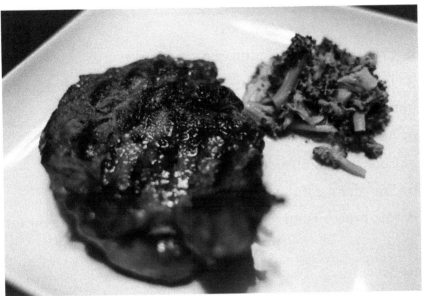

Serving: 4

Prep Time: 5 minutes

Cook Time: 15 minutes

Ingredients

- 4 ounces butter
- ¾ pound Ribeye steak, sliced
- 9 ounces broccoli, chopped
- 1 yellow onion, sliced
- 1 tablespoon coconut aminos
- 1 tablespoon pumpkin seeds
- Salt and pepper to taste

How To

1. Slice steak and the onions

2. Chop broccoli, including the stem parts

3. Take a frying pan and place it over medium heat, add butter and let it melt

4. Add meat and season accordingly with salt and pepper

5. Cook until both sides are browned

6. Transfer meat to platter

7. Add broccoli and onion to the frying pan, add more butter if needed

8. Brown

9. Add coconut aminos and return the meat

10. Stir and season again

11. Serve with a dollop of butter with a sprinkle of pumpkin seeds

12. Enjoy!

Nutrition (Per Serving)

- Calories: 875
- Fat: 75g
- Carbohydrates: 8g
- Protein: 40g

29. Cilantro And Lime Skirt Steak

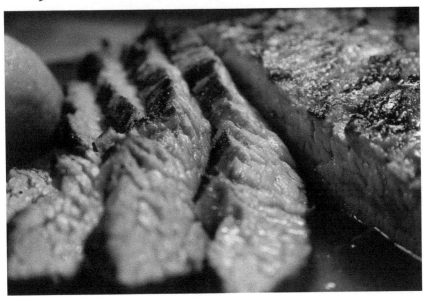

Serving: 3

Prep Time: 45 minutes

Cook Time: 10 minutes

<u>**Ingredients**</u>

For the Cilantro Lime Steak Marinade

- 1 pound of Skirt Steak
- ¼ cup of coconut aminos
- ¼ cup of Olive Oil
- 1 medium sized lime, juiced
- 1 teaspoon of garlic, minced
- 1 small sized Handful Cilantro

- ¼ teaspoon of Red Pepper Flakes

For the Cilantro Paste

- 1 teaspoon of garlic, minced
- ½ a teaspoon of Salt
- 1 cup of lightly fresh cilantro
- ¼ cup of olive oil
- ½ a medium sized lemon, juiced
- 1 medium sized deseeded Jalapeno
- ½ a teaspoon of Cumin
- ½ a teaspoon of Coriander

How To

1. Remove the outer silver skin off the skirt steak
2. Take a plastic bag and add the Cilantro Lime Steak marinade ingredients to the bag, add the steak and mix to coat it up
3. Allow it to marinate for 45 minutes in your fridge
4. Make the sauce by adding the paste ingredients to a food processor and pulse until blended to a paste
5. Take an iron skillet and place it over medium-high heat
6. Remove the steak from the bag transfer steak to the pan and sear both sides (each side for 2-3 minutes)
7. Serve with the cilantro sauce on top
8. Enjoy!

Nutrition(Per Serving)

- Calories: 432
- Fat: 32g
- Carbohydrates: 4g
- Protein: 38g

30. Mushroom And Olive "Mediterranean" Steak

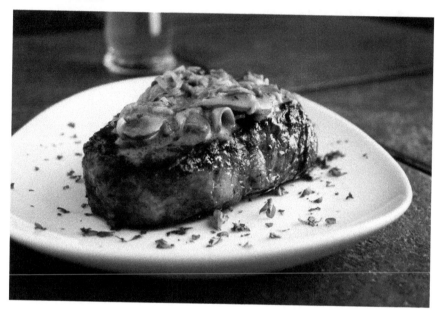

Serving: 4

Prep Time: 10 minutes

Cook Time: 14 minutes

Ingredients

- 1 pound boneless beef sirloin steak, ¾ inch thick, cut into 4 pieces
- 1 large red onion, chopped
- 1 cup mushrooms
- 4 garlic cloves, thinly sliced
- 4 tablespoons olive oil

73

- ½ cup green olives, coarsely chopped
- 1 cup parsley leaves, finely cut

How To

1. Take a large sized skillet and place it over medium high heat
2. Add oil and let it heat p
3. Add beef and cook until both sides are browned, remove beef and drain fat
4. Add rest of the oil to skillet and heat I up
5. Add onions, garlic and cook for 2-3 minutes
6. Stir well
7. Add mushrooms olives and cook until mushrooms are thoroughly done
8. Return beef to skillet and lower heat to medium
9. Cook for 3-4 minutes (covered_
10. Stir in parsley
11. Serve and enjoy!

Nutrition (Per Serving)

- Calories: 386
- Fat: 30g
- Carbohydrates: 11g
- Protein: 21g

31.Satisfying Low-Carb Beef Liver Salad

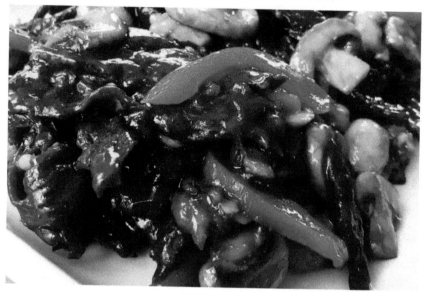

Serving: 3

Prep Time: 10 minutes

Cook Time: Nil

Ingredients

- 3-4 ounces beef liver, cooked
- 1 egg, hard boiled
- 1 ounce dried mushroom
- 1 whole onion, minced
- 2 ounces mayonnaise
- 2 ounces olive oil
- Salt and pepper to taste

- Dill for serving
- ½ a red bell pepper, sliced

How To

1. Cut mushroom and livers into stripsand transfer to a bowl
2. Peel the egg and slice it, transfer to bowl
3. Add remaining ingredients and toss well
4. Sprinkle with dill and serve!

Nutrition (Per Serving)

- Calories: 300
- Fat: 26g
- Carbohydrates: 5g
- Protein: 10g

Perfect Aromatic Beef Roast

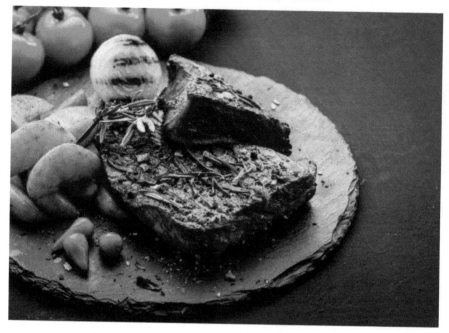

Serving: 4

Prep Time: 10 minutes

Cook Time: 50 minutes

Ingredients

- 1 lb of beef sirloin or similar lean cut for roast
- 2 tbsp of mustard
- 2 tbsp of olive oil
- 2 tbsp of garlic salt
- 1 spring of fresh rosemary

How To

1. Combine the mustard, olive oil, and garlic salt in a small bowl.

2. Take the roast beef, remove excess fat and make small incisions lengthwise so you can let the mixture penetrate more easily.

3. Brush the mustard mixture over the beef, making sure it all nicely coated.

4. Place on a baking dish and arrange the rosemary leaves on the sides for extra aroma.

5. Cook in a preheated oven at 380F/180 C for 50 minutes (for a medium cook inside).

6. Serve with mashed sweet potatoes and/or salad

Nutrition (Per Serving)

- Calories: 646
- Fat: 27g
- Carbohydrates: 0.1g
- Protein: 96g

33. Beef Packed Zucchini Boats

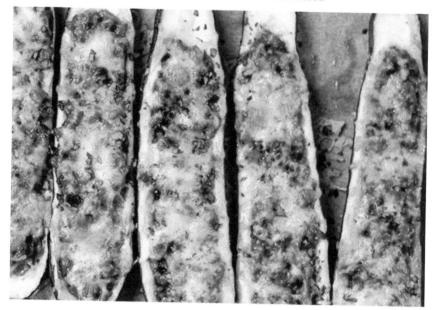

Serving: 4

Prep Time: 10 minutes

Cook Time: 30 minutes

Ingredients

- 1 lb of ground beef with around 80% meat and 20% fat ratio
- 1 cup of red Mexican salsa
- 4 medium zucchinis
- 1/2 shredded cheddar cheese
- 1 tbsp of olive oil

How To

1. Take the zucchinis, cut in half lengthwise, and scoop out the middle flesh inside (leaving enough flesh to make a boat on the sides). Take a form and pinch the insides slightly.

2. Heat the pan with olive oil and add the ground beef.

3. Sauté for 7-8 minutes or until most of the juices have evaporated.

4. Add the salsa and cook for another couple of minutes

5. Distribute the ground beef and salsa over the zucchini boats

6. Sprinkle with the cheese on top of each.

7. Bake in the oven for 15 minutes and serve

Nutrition (Per Serving)

- Calories: 280
- Fat: 13g
- Carbohydrates: 4.2g
- Protein: 30g

34.   Spicy Chipotle Steak

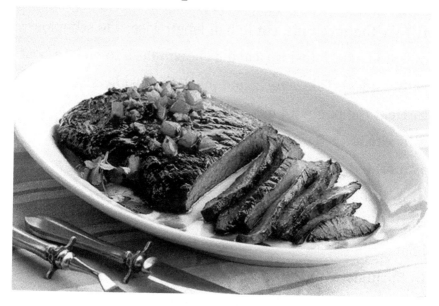

Serving: 4

Prep Time: 10 minutes

Cook Time: 10-20 minutes

Ingredients

- 2 sirloin steaks, cut into thin strips
- 1 tbsp of chipotle seasoning powder
- 2 tbsp of olive oil
- 1/4 cup tomato paste
- Salt to taste

How To

1. Combine the tomato paste, olive oil, and chipotle seasoning with salt to make a marinade.

2. Brush the mixture onto the steaks.

3. Heat a grilling pan and cook the steaks 2-3 minutes on each side for medium inside or depending on how cooked you want them to be

Nutrition (Per Serving)

- Calories: 470
- Fat: 24g
- Carbohydrates: 4g
- Protein: 50g

35.   Beef Cheeseburger Wraps

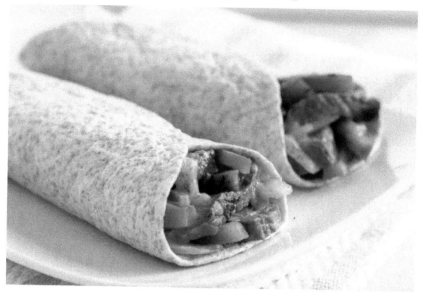

Serving: 4

Prep Time: 10 minutes

Cook Time: 50 minutes

<u>Ingredients</u>

- 8 oz. of ground beef with 20% fat
- ¹/4 cup chopped onion
- 4 small low carb tortillas
- 2 slices of mild cheddar cheese
- 2 tbsp of salsa

How To

1. Lightly grease a pan and add the onion and saute for a couple of minutes until almost transparent.

2. Add the ground beef and sauté for 4-5 minutes or until the juices have evaporated.

3. Add the salsa and toss.

4. Distribute the ground beef mixture onto the tortilla chips and top with parmesan cheese.

5. Serve optionally with a bit of sour cream

Nutrition (Per Serving)

- Calories: 456
- Fat: 21g
- Carbohydrates: 5g
- Protein: 37g

36.   Cheddar Jalapeno Meatloaf

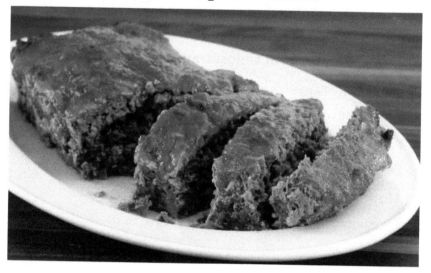

Serving: 4

Prep Time: 10 minutes

Cook Time: 35-40 minutes

Ingredients

- 2 lb ground beef
- ½ tsp cumin
- 2 jalapenos, sliced
- 1 1/2 tbsp of garlic salt
- 1 ½ cups of cheddar cheese

How To

1. Preheat the oven to 375F/180C.

2. Combine all the ingredients together except the jalapenos and cheese.

3. Fill a deep baking dish (around 8X8 inches) with the ground beef and spice mixture, top with the jalapenos, and finish with the layer of cheddar cheese.

4. Bake in the oven for 35-40 minutes. Let rest for 5 minutes before serving and cut ideally into squares or triangles before serving

Nutrition (Per Serving)

- Calories: 407
- Fat: 28g
- Carbohydrates: 2.3g
- Protein: 30g

37. Perfect Philly Cheesesteak Stuffed Peppers

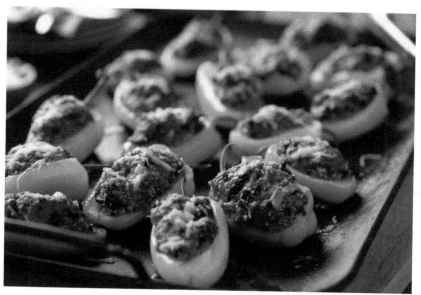

Serving: 4

Prep Time: 10 minutes

Cook Time: 20 minutes

Ingredients

- 2 large bell peppers cut in half lengthwise
- 8 oz. of thinly sliced roast beef or pastrami beef
- 6 oz. of baby mushrooms, sliced
- 8 slices of provolone or cheddar cheese
- 2 tbsp of salted butter

How To

1. Make sure that the bell peppers are cut lengthwise into halves and contain no seeds.

2. In a pan, melt the butter and add the mushrooms. Saute for 3-4 minutes and remove from the heat.

3. Take the bell pepper halves and start arranging one slice of cheese over the bottom layer of the pepper, then 2 slices of pastrami on each, and then a few mushrooms. Finish off each pepper boat with an extra slice of cheese on top.

4. In a preheated oven (around 400F/200C), pop the peppers and cook for 18-20 minutes so that the peppers are cooked, and the cheese is melted.

5. Let cool for 5 minutes and serve

Nutrition (Per Serving)

- Calories: 458
- Fat: 36g
- Carbohydrates: 8g
- Protein: 27g

38.   Grilled Beef Short Loin

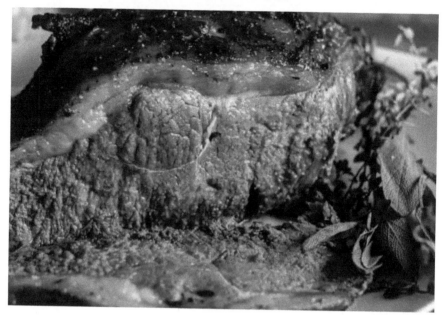

Serving: 4

Prep Time: 10 minutes

Cook Time: 15-20 minutes

<u>Ingredients</u>

- 1 1/2 pounds beef short loin
- 2 thyme sprigs, chopped
- 1 rosemary sprig, chopped
- 1 teaspoon garlic powder
- Sea salt and ground black pepper, to taste

How To

1. Place all of the above ingredients in a re-sealable zipper bag. Shake until the short beef loin is well coated on all sides.

2. Cook on a preheated grill for 15 to 20 minutes, flipping once or twice during the cooking time.

3. Let it stand for 5 minutes before slicing and serving.

Nutrition (Per Serving)

- Calories: 313
- Fat: 11g
- Carbohydrates: 0.1g
- Protein: 52g

39.   Hearty Beef Bourguignon

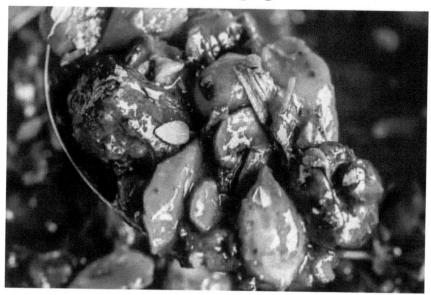

Serving: 4

Prep Time: 10 minutes

Cook Time: 60-70 minutes

Ingredients

- 1 1/2 pounds shoulder steak, cut into cubes
- 1 tablespoon Herbs de Provence
- 1 onion, chopped
- 1 celery stalk, chopped
- 1 cup red Burgundy wine

How To

1. Heat up a lightly greased soup pot over a medium-high flame. Now brown the beef in batches until no longer pink.
2. Add a splash of wine to deglaze your pan.
3. Add the Herbs de Provence, onion, celery, and wine to the pot; pour in 3 cups of water and stir to combine well. Bring to a rapid boil; then, turn the heat to medium-low.
4. Cover and let it simmer for 1 hour 10 minutes. Serve over hot cauliflower rice if desired. Enjoy!

Nutrition (Per Serving)

- Calories: 217
- Fat: 4g
- Carbohydrates: 4g
- Protein: 0.4g

40. Zucchini And Cheddar Beef Mugs

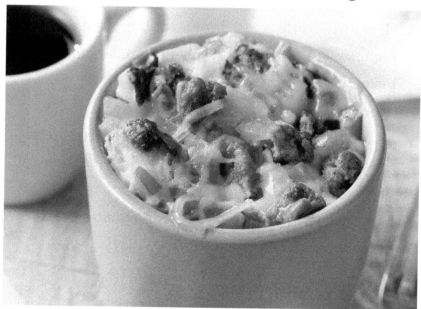

Serving: 4

Prep Time: 10 minutes

Cook Time: 5 minutes

<u>Ingredients</u>

- 4 oz roast beef deli slices, torn apart
- 3 tbsp sour cream
- 1 small zucchini, chopped
- 2 tbsp chopped green chilies
- 3 oz shredded cheddar cheese

How To

1. Divide the beef slices at the bottom of 2 wide mugs and spread 1 tbsp of sour cream.
2. Top with 2 zucchini slices, season with salt and pepper, add green chilies, top with the remaining sour cream, and then cheddar cheese.
3. Place the mugs in the microwave for 1-2 minutes until the cheese melts.
4. Remove the mugs, let cool for 1 minute, and serve.

Nutrition (Per Serving)

- Calories: 188
- Fat: 9g
- Carbohydrates: 4g
- Protein: 18g

41. Beef Stuffed Peppers

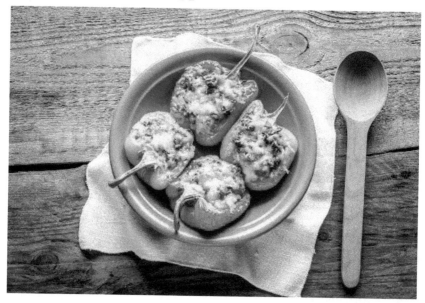

Serving: 4

Prep Time: 10 minutes

Cook Time: 50 minutes

Ingredients

- 1 /2-pound ground beef
- 1 garlic clove, minced
- Sea salt and ground black pepper, to taste
- 1/4 cup cream of onion soup
- 1/2 teaspoon paprika

How To

1. Heat the olive oil in a saute pan over moderate heat. Once hot, sear the ground beef for 5 to 6 minutes, turning once or twice to ensure even cooking.

2. Add in the cream of onion soup, paprika, salt, and black pepper. Cook for a further 3 minutes until heated through. The meat thermometer should register 145 degrees F.

3. Serve in individual plates garnished with freshly snipped chives if desired. Enjoy!

Nutrition (Per Serving)

- Calories: 395
- Fat: 24g
- Carbohydrates: 0.8g
- Protein: 40g

42.   Fine Filet Mignon In Dijon Sauce

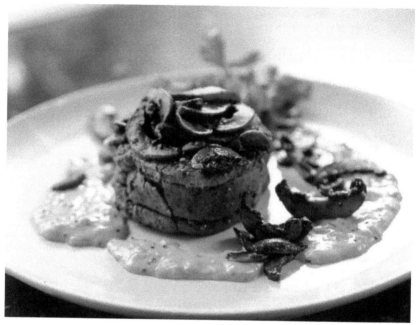

Serving: 4

Prep Time: 10 minutes

Cook Time: 10-15 minutes

<u>Ingredients</u>

- 2 teaspoons lard, at room temperature
- 2 pounds beef filet mignon, cut into bite-sized chunks
- Flaky salt and ground black pepper, to season
- 1 tablespoon Dijon mustard
- 1 cup double cream

How To

1. Melt the lard in a saucepan over moderate heat; now, sear the filet mignon for 2 to 3 minutes per side—season with salt and pepper to taste.
2. Fold in the Dijon mustard and cream. Reduce the heat to medium-low and continue to cook for a further 6 minutes or until the sauce has reduced slightly.
3. Serve in individual plates, garnished with cauli rice if desired. Enjoy!

Nutrition (Per Serving)

- Calories: 301
- Fat: 2g
- Carbohydrates: 2g
- Protein: 34g

43.   Shitake Butter Beef Dish

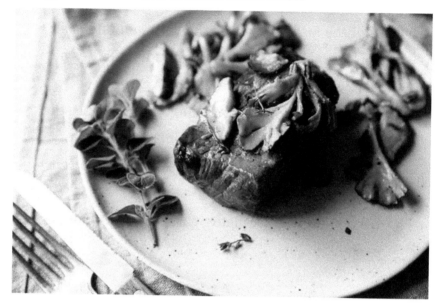

Serving: 4

Prep Time: 10 minutes

Cook Time: 5-10 minutes

Ingredients

- 2 cups shitake mushrooms, sliced
- 4 ribeye steaks
- 2 tbsp butter
- 2 tsp olive oil
- Salt and black pepper to taste

How To

1. Heat olive oil in a pan over medium heat. Rub the steaks with salt and pepper and cook for 4 minutes per side. Set aside.
2. Melt butter in the pan and cook the shitakes for 4 minutes.
3. Pour the butter and mushrooms over the steak.

Nutrition (Per Serving)

- Calories: 307
- Fat: 31g
- Carbohydrates: 3g
- Protein: 33g

44.   Crazy Beef Meatballs

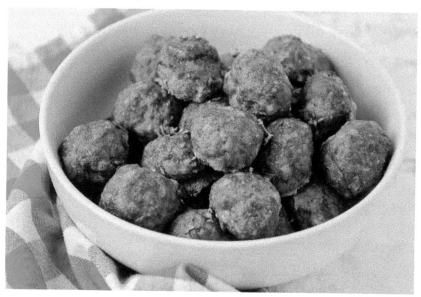

Serving: 4

Prep Time: 10 minutes

Cook Time: 18-20 minutes

Ingredients

- 1 lb ground beef
- ¹/2 cup grated parmesan cheese
- 1 tbsp minced garlic (or paste)
- ¹/2 cup mozzarella cheese
- 1 tsp freshly ground pepper

How To

1. Preheat your oven to 400°F/200°C.

2. In a bowl, mix all the ingredients together.

3. Roll the meat mixture into 6 generous meatballs.

4. Bake inside your oven at 170°F/80°C for about 18 minutes.

5. Serve with sauce!

Nutrition (Per Serving)

- Calories: 380
- Fat: 22g
- Carbohydrates: 1g
- Protein: 18g

45.   Delicious Beef Casserole

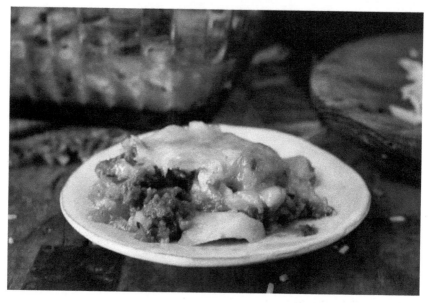

Serving: 4

Prep Time: 10 minutes

Cook Time: 30-40 minutes

Ingredients

- $1/2$ lb. ground beef
- $1/2$ cup chopped onion
- $1/2$ bag coleslaw mix
- 1-1/2 cups tomato sauce
- 1 tbsp lemon juice

How To

1. In a skillet, cook the ground beef until browned and to the side.
2. Mix in the onion and cabbage to the skillet and sauté until soft.
3. Add the ground beef back in along with the tomato sauce and lemon juice.
4. Bring the mixture to a boil, then cover and simmer for 30 minutes.
5. Enjoy!

Nutrition (Per Serving)

- Calories: 275
- Fat: 20g
- Carbohydrates: 6g
- Protein: 20g

46.   Ground Beef Hamburger Patties

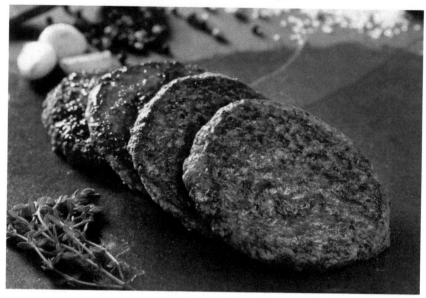

Serving: 4

Prep Time: 10 minutes

Cook Time: 5-10 minutes

<u>Ingredients</u>

- ½ *an* egg
- 12 oz. ground beef
- 1and 1/2 oz. crumbled feta cheese
- 1 oz. butter
- Salt & Black pepper

How To

1. In a mixing bowl, add the feta cheese, ground beef, black pepper, egg, and salt, then mix to combine well.
2. Shape the mixture into equal patties.
3. Put a pan on fire to melt the butter.
4. Cook the patties for 4 minutes on each side on medium-low heat.
5. Serve!

Nutrition (Per Serving)

- Calories: 488
- Fat: 27g
- Carbohydrates: 2g
- Protein: 56g

47.   Creative Lamb Chops

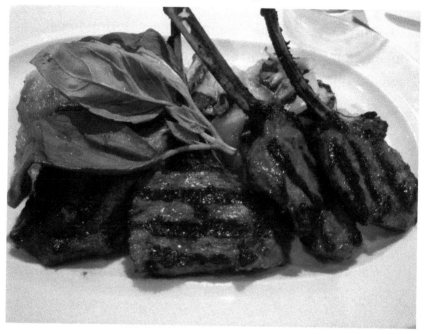

Serving: 3

Prep Time: 35 minutes

Cook Time: 5 minutes

<u>Ingredients</u>

- ¼ cup olive oil
- ¼ cup mint, fresh and chopped
- 8 lamb rib chops
- 1 tablespoon garlic, minced
- 1 tablespoon rosemary, fresh and chopped

How To

1. Add rosemary, garlic, mint, olive oil into a bowl and mix well

2. Keep a tablespoon of the mixture on the side for later use

3. Toss lamb chops into the marinade, letting them marinate for 30 minutes

4. Take a cast iron skillet and place it over medium-high heat

5. Add lamb and cook for 2 minutes per side for medium rare

6. Let the lamb rest for a few minutes and drizzle remaining marinade

7. Serve and enjoy!

Nutrition (Per Serving)

- Calories: 566
- Fat: 40g
- Carbohydrates: 2g
- Protein: 47g

48.   Crazy Lamb Salad

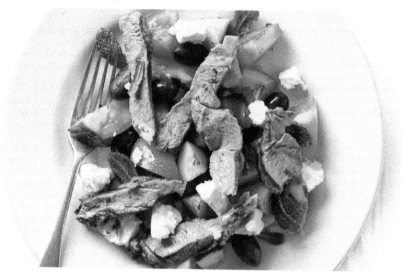

Serving: 4

Prep Time: 10 minutes

Cook Time: 35 minutes

<u>Ingredients</u>

- 1 tablespoon olive oil
- 3 pounds leg of lamb, bone removed, leg butterflied
- Salt and pepper to taste
- 1 teaspoon cumin
- Pinch of dried thyme
- 2 garlic cloves, peeled and minced

For Salad

- 4 ounces feta cheese, crumbled
- ½ cup pecans
- 2 cups spinach
- 1 and ½ tablespoons lemon juice
- ¼ cup olive oil
- 1 cup fresh mint, chopped

How To

1. Rub lamb with salt and pepper, 1 tablespoon oil, thyme, cumin, minced garlic

2. Pre-heat your grill to medium-high h and transfer lamb

3. Cook for 40 minutes, making sure to flip it once

4. Take a lined baking sheet and spread pecans

5. Toast in oven for 10 minutes at 350 degree F

6. Transfer grilled lamb to cutting board and let it cool

7. Slice

8. Take a salad bowl and add spinach, 1 cup mint, feta cheese, ¼ cup olive oil, lemon juice, toasted pecans, salt, pepper and toss well

9. Add lamb slices on top

10. Serve and enjoy!

Nutrition (Per Serving)

- Calories: 334
- Fat: 33g
- Carbohydrates: 5g
- Protein: 7g

49.   Healthy Slow-Cooker Lamb Leg

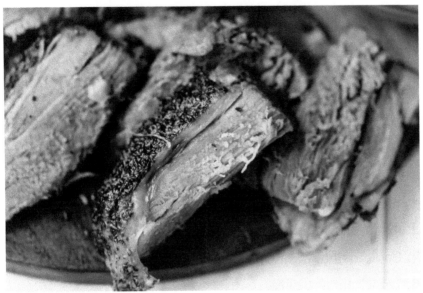

Serving: 6

Prep Time: 10 minutes

Cook Time: 8 hours

Ingredients

- 2 pounds lamb leg
- Salt and pepper to taste
- 1 tablespoon vanilla bean extract
- 2 tablespoons mustard
- ¼ cup olive oil
- 4 thyme sprigs
- 6 mint leaves

- 1 teaspoon garlic, minced
- Pinch of dried rosemary

How To

1. Add oil to your Slow Cooker

2. Add lamb, salt, pepper, vanilla bean extract, mustard, rosemary, garlic to your Slow Cooker and rub the mixture well

3. Place lid and cook on LOW for 7 hours

4. Add mint and thyme

5. Cook for 1 hour more

6. Let it cool and slice

7. Serve with pan juices

8. Enjoy!

Nutrition (Per Serving)

- Calories: 400
- Fat: 34g
- Carbohydrates: 3g
- Protein: 26g

50. Spicy Paprika Lamb Chops

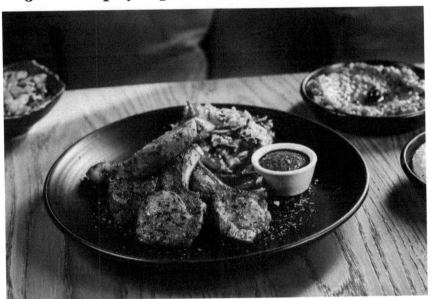

Serving: 4

Prep Time: 10 minutes

Cook Time: 15 minutes

Ingredients

- 2 lamb racks, cut into chops
- Salt and pepper to taste
- 3 tablespoons paprika
- ¾ cup cumin powder
- 1 teaspoon chili powder

How To

1. Take a bowl and add paprika, cumin, chili, salt, pepper and stir

2. Add lamb chops and rub the mixture

3. Heat grill over medium-temperature and add lamb chops, cook for 5 minutes

4. Flip and cook for 5 minutes more, flip again

5. Cook for 2 minutes, flip and cook for 2 minutes more

6. Serve and enjoy!

Nutrition (Per Serving)

- Calories: 200
- Fat: 5g
- Carbohydrates: 4g
- Protein: 8g

Lightning Source UK Ltd.
Milton Keynes UK
UKHW020711300721
388030UK00005B/68